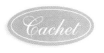

Pampering
Pedicure

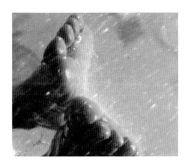

TOP THAT!

Copyright © 2004 Top That! Publishing plc,
Top That! Publishing, 25031 W. Avenue Stanford, Suite #60, Valencia, CA 91355
www.topthatpublishing.com

Contents

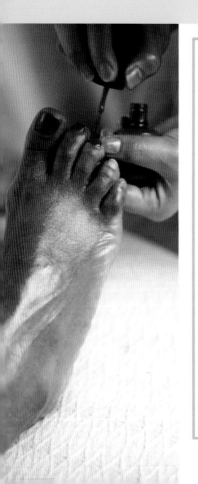

Introduction

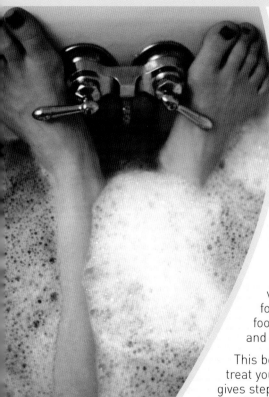

Our feet are one of the hardest working parts of our body, yet they are often the most neglected. They carry us wherever we go, and yet we abuse them on a daily basis. Often the only time we think about them is when we kick off our shoes at the end of a tiring day and "put our feet up."

Healthy feet contribute to your overall well-being and comfort; remember how good it feels when you go barefoot on vacation. Treating yourself to a foot massage, pedicure or other foot treatment makes you feel good and indeed **IS** good for you.

This book will explain why you should treat your feet, and how to do it. It even gives step-by-step instructions for some home treatments that will make your feet love you.

What are feet?

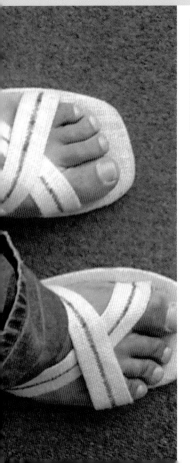

The first humans became upright about one million years ago. This freed our hands for more intricate tasks—the start of civilization. However, standing on just two feet doubled the load on them, and shoes were required to protect them from injury and cold.

Complex feet

Our feet are strong and flexible. Although relatively small compared with the rest of our body, each foot contains 26 bones (together our feet contain a quarter of the bones in our body), 33 joints and more than 100 tendons, muscles and ligaments, as well as nerves and blood vessels.

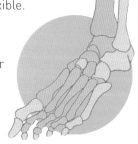

Tough skin

The skin on our feet is some of the toughest anywhere on the body, particularly on the balls of the foot and on the heels where most of the load of walking is borne.

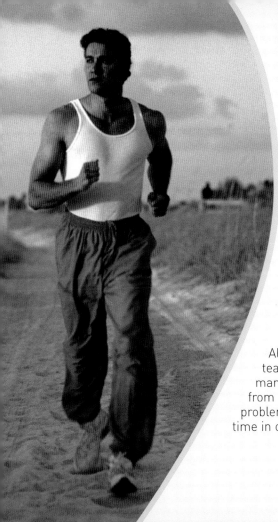

Left or right footed

As people can be left-handed or right-handed, they can also be right- or left-footed. Try to kick with each of your feet and you will see just how much foot coordination we take for granted every day.

What do feet do?

Our feet help us walk, run and jump, and act as shock absorbers with each step we take. They protect other joints in our legs, hips and back. The average person take 8,000 to 10,000 steps a day and walks 115,000 miles in their lifetime—the equivalent of walking four times around Earth!

All this makes for a lot of wear and tear on our feet, so it is no wonder many of us suffer from foot problems at some time in our lives.

Superstitions and customs

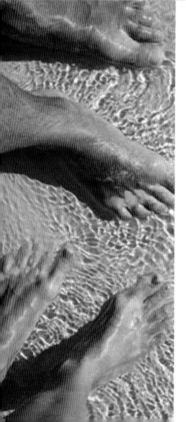

There are many superstitions and customs surrounding feet and shoes.

Weddings

Many wedding customs involve shoes. It is thought that shoes bring good luck. Instead of throwing her bouquet, a bride throws one of her shoes. As the happy couple leave the wedding reception, guests throw shoes at them to ensure good luck. It is considered extra lucky if either the couple or their carriage are hit!

Lucky shoes

In the Philippines it is bad luck to give someone a pair of shoes or slippers unless the recipient pays something for them—even one cent is enough. Old shoes were considered a good luck token, and even today many people still wear them on Friday 13th.

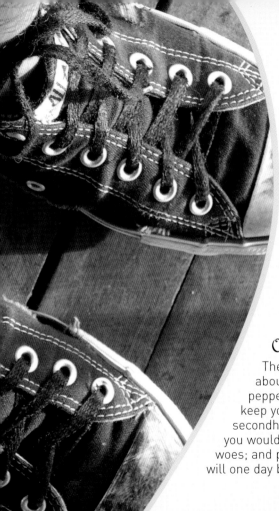

Left foot fear

Bad luck has always been associated with the left foot. Putting the left foot out of bed first in the morning would ensure an unlucky day! In ancient Greece, men embarking on a hazardous journey would often wear a shoe on their right foot and keep their left foot bare.

Pagan times

In pagan times, coming upon a person who was barefoot, especially in the morning, was considered bad luck. Meeting a person who was flat-footed or splay-footed was a particularly bad omen.

Old wives' tales

There are also many old wives' tales about feet, such as: if you put a red pepper in your shoes in winter it will keep your feet warm; accepting secondhand shoes will bring bad luck as you would walk in the former owner's woes; and people with holes in their shoes will one day become rich.

7

Footcare tips

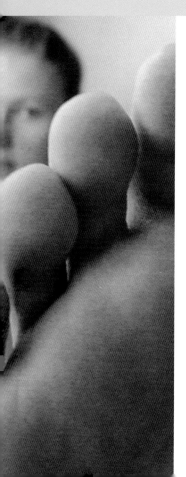

As the saying goes "Care for your feet and they will care for you." Our modern lifestyle of pounding hard sidewalks, increasing obesity (the extra weight puts more strain on the feet) and wearing unsuitable footwear has taken its toll on our feet. Caring for your feet daily and the prompt treatment of ailments are essential for your health. Here are some tips for keeping your feet happy and healthy!

Foot pain

Foot pain is not normal, so don't ignore it. Pain is distinct from the normal aches that a long day can provoke in our feet. Many conditions can be cured, so go to see a chiropodist or podiatrist if the pain persists.

Washing

Wash your feet daily, but don't soak them as this can result in excessive dryness. Use a gentle soap that will not strip the oils from the delicate skin on your feet.

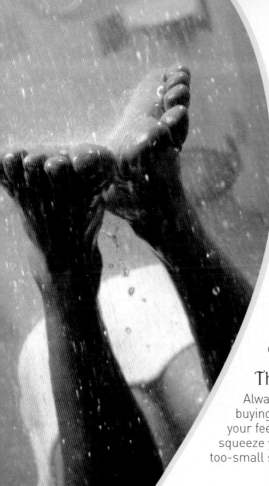

Rinsing

Rinse off soap and dry thoroughly, especially between your toes.

Hard skin

Gently remove any hard skin, using a pumice stone or skin file when the skin is softened after bathing. Never rub over a joint.

Foot inspection

Inspect your feet regularly. Take note of any changes in color and temperature. Look at your toenails for thickening or discoloration (a sign of fungus). Growths such as corns, calluses and warts should be treated by a footcare specialist or doctor.

The right shoes

Always wear well-fitting shoes. When buying shoes it is a good idea to have your feet measured properly. Don't try to squeeze your feet into the pair of one-size-too-small shoes that you really want!

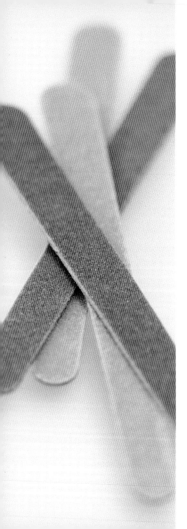

Footcare dos

When wearing sandals or when sunbathing always remember to put sunblock on your feet.

Wear clean socks or stockings daily and make sure that they are the correct size. Socks and stockings appear to be soft and stretchy, but if they are too small the stretched fabric can put considerable strain on your feet.

Use home remedies for corns and warts with care as they may cause damage to the surrounding skin. More severe infections should always be treated with proper medicine obtained from a pharmacy, or on the advice of a doctor, podiatrist or a chiropodist.

The best form of exercise for your feet is walking, so walk as much as you can. Like any other part of your body, the muscles in your feet get fitter and more flexible the more you use them.

Rest any injury to your foot immediately. Injuries, such as sprains and pulled muscles, can be made worse very quickly if you continue to put weight on the injured foot.

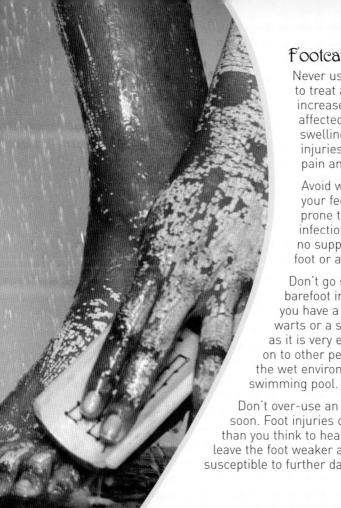

Footcare don'ts ⊗

Never use heat or hot water to treat a foot injury—heat increases blood flow to the affected area, causing swelling. Treat minor injuries with ice to reduce pain and swelling.

Avoid walking barefoot— your feet will be more prone to injury and infections and there is no support for either your foot or ankle.

Don't go swimming or barefoot in a public place if you have a foot infection, warts or a similar problem, as it is very easy to pass these on to other people, especially in the wet environment of a swimming pool.

Don't over-use an injured foot too soon. Foot injuries can take longer than you think to heal properly and often leave the foot weaker and more susceptible to further damage.

Footwear

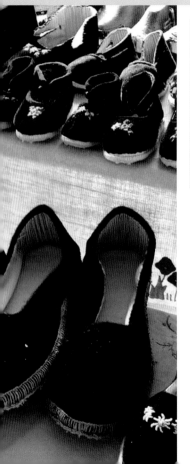

People have worn shoes for thousands of years. The earliest type of footwear was probably made of weaved grass or rawhide held on the foot with thongs. The main function of these simple sandals was to protect the feet from the cold and injury. Although this is still the case, today's shoes are also fashion accessories and statements, and many of the shoes that we wear today do more harm to our feet than good.

Modern shoes

In our modern, busy lifestyle, our feet take a real hammering. Walking on hard surfaces, like concrete, is very jolting on our feet.

In addition to this, more of us are overweight, which puts added strain on our joints.

Around 80 percent of foot problems occur in women—wearing high heels is often the root cause of these.

Footwear has recently become more and more specialized and now there is a shoe for almost every conceivable need and activity.

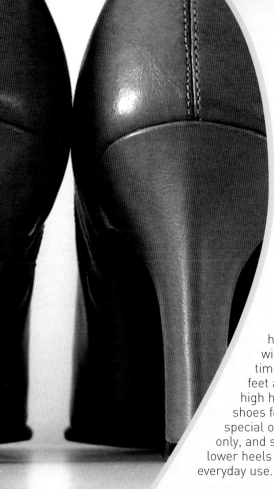

High heel horror

Despite the fact that women love to wear high heels, they are the cause of many foot problems.

High heels can cause calluses from the shoe rubbing on the bone, bunions and nerve problems to our feet.

They are also responsible for knee and back problems, shortened calf muscles and injuries from falls.

Although you might not be prepared to give up your high heels completely, it is wise to limit the amount of time you wear them to give your feet a break. Think of those extra high heels as shoes for a special occasion only, and stick to lower heels for everyday use.

Choosing the right shoes for you

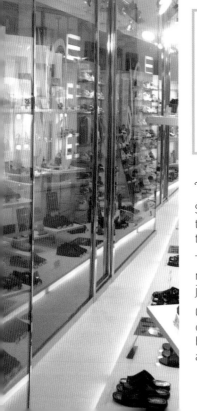

Choosing footwear is not only important for protection and style, but also for the health of our feet. The wrong shoes can cause foot ailments or make existing ones worse.

The best time to shop for shoes is in the afternoon, as your feet tend to swell slightly during the day. Have your feet measured every time you buy a pair of shoes.

The art of choosing

Shoes made of leather are best for your feet as they allow them to "breathe," and stretch to mold to the shape of your foot.

The sole of the shoe should be strong, flexible and non-slip, while a thick insole will cushion your joints from the jarring effects of walking.

Often, a more expensive shoe will well outlast a cheaper pair, making them better value in the long run, as well as probably being better fitting and more comfortable.

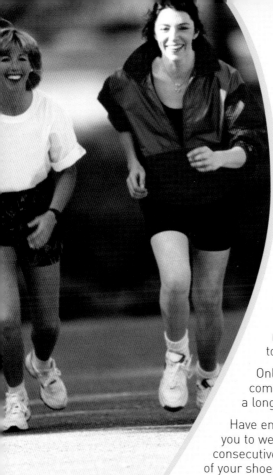

Remember, when choosing:

High heels and pointed shoes pinch the toes and push your center of gravity forward, leading to poor posture.

Opt for shoes that are designed for the activity you will be doing. Aerobics shoes for aerobics, walking shoes for walking, for example.

Try new shoes on both feet. Many people have one foot larger than the other, so buy shoes to fit your largest foot.

There should be enough room in the shoe for all your toes to be able to wriggle.

Only buy shoes that feel comfortable and wear them in over a long period of time.

Have enough pairs of shoes to allow you to wear different shoes on consecutive days. This will let the inside of your shoes to dry out properly, making them healthier to wear.

Feet facts and figures

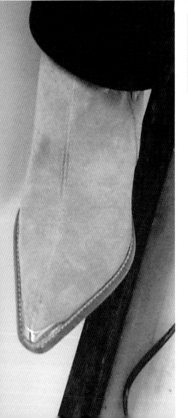

Need to know a bit more about your feet? The following facts and figures will help you realize how complex and hard working your feet can be!

That's amazing!

Your toes take half of your body's weight every time you lift your heels off the ground when you are walking.

There are around 250,000 sweat glands in your feet, and you can lose up to 16 oz of perspiration through each foot every day.

The many simple joints in your feet enable a wide degree of flexibility.

Each step you take exerts a pressure on your feet three to four times that of your body weight. When you run, this rises to seven times!

Toenails only grow at around half the speed of fingernails. A lost toenail will take between six and nine months to regrow completely.

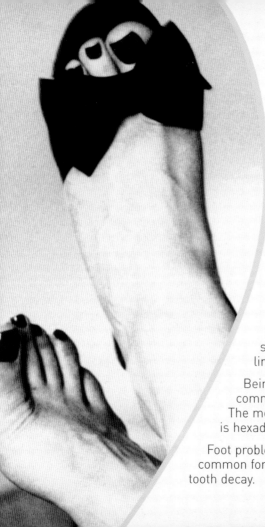

Your feet mirror your general health. Early symptoms of conditions such as diabetes, arthritis, nerve and circulatory disorders can often be shown in the feet.

Minor foot ailments may be the first sign of a serious health problem.

Babies' feet grow quickly and will reach almost half their adult size in the first year of life.

Your big toe is vital in maintaining a sense of balance. If you lose your big toe it becomes almost impossible to walk in a straight line without a path or line to follow.

Being born with six toes is more common than you might think. The medical term for this extra toe is hexadactyly.

Foot problems are the third most common form of illness behind colds and tooth decay.

17

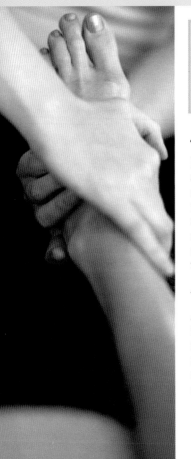

The foot is a complicated and delicate part of our bodies. It is no wonder that things can go wrong. Indeed, over 90 percent of us will suffer from a foot ailment at some time in our lives!

Athlete's foot

In spite of the name, anyone can suffer from athlete's foot. Athlete's foot is a fungal infection causing burning, itching, cracking and blisters, most commonly between the toes, but it can appear anywhere on the foot. There may also be some associated swelling. The infection may subside after a while but it will not disappear without proper treatment.

Treatment

Antifungal powder or cream is the basis of the treatment. Remember to dry your feet thoroughly after bathing and wear cotton socks to absorb moisture. Athlete's foot fungus is very contagious so it is important not to share a towel with anyone until the infection has been completely eliminated.

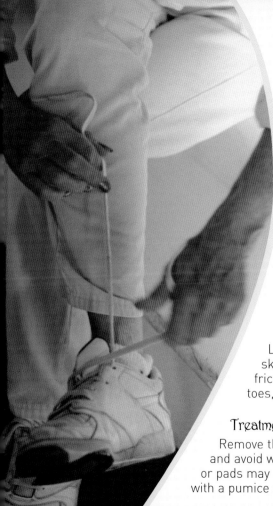

Blisters

Blisters are caused by friction when the skin becomes hot and sweaty and rubs against your shoe. Fluid builds up between the layers of skin in the affected area, forming a raised bump.

Treatment

Most blisters heal if left alone. Never pop a blister as it will be more likely to become infected. Keep the area clean and dry and avoid pressure or rubbing on it while it is healing. Seek medical attention if there is any sign of infection.

Calluses

Like a corn, a callus is an area of skin that thickens due to repeated friction. They are usually found on toes, heels and the soles of the feet.

Treatment

Remove the cause, such as ill-fitting shoes, and avoid wearing high heels. Shoe cushions or pads may be helpful, as is gentle rubbing with a pumice stone.

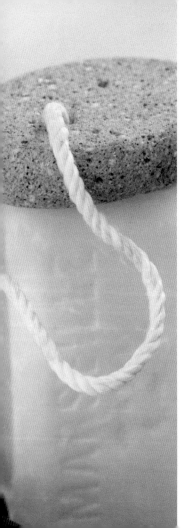

Corns

A corn is an area of thickened skin caused by repeated pressure or rubbing and is commonly found on the tops or sides of the toes. Corns are painful when pressed.

Treatment

Remove the cause, which is usually ill-fitting shoes. The corn can be protected with a corn pad. Gentle rubbing with a pumice stone will wear the hard skin down. Corn removing solutions can be quite acidic and irritating to sensitive skin. They should only be used with care and never by people suffering from diabetes.

Ingrown toenails

If not infected, soak the foot in warm water and apply a mild antiseptic lotion. When cutting toenails, don't cut them too short and always cut the nail straight across. If any infection is present, consult a doctor. An ingrown toenail can be extremely painful and, unless treated, an infection can easily spread, leading to much more serious problems.

Treatment

Remove the cause, such as ill-fitting shoes and avoid wearing high heels. Shoe cushions or pads may be helpful, as well as gentle rubbing with a pumice stone. If the nail is extremely bad, surgery may be needed to fully correct the problem.

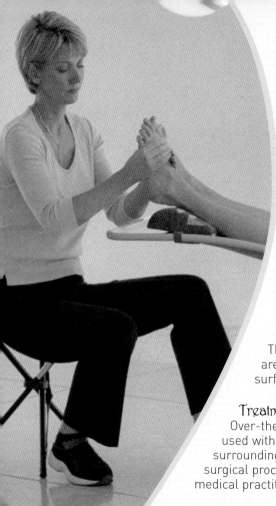

Bunions

The joints of the big toe become misaligned, with the first joint slanting outwards and the second angled towards the other toes, sometimes resting over or under the second toe. The toe may become very painful, with swelling and inflammation around the area.

Treatment

Well-fitting shoes with a wide toe area can provide some relief. Bunion shields or bandages can be applied. If severe, consult your doctor.

Plantar warts

These are caused by a virus and are hard and flat with a rough surface. They may be painful.

Treatment

Over-the-counter remedies should be used with care as they can damage the surrounding healthy tissue. Simple surgical procedures can be performed by a medical practitioner or a chiropodist.

21

Toenail care

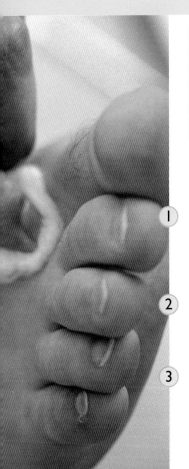

Beautiful feet need beautiful nails. Clean, well-tended nails not only make your feet look fantastic, they are necessary to maintain healthy feet. It doesn't take long to transform dull, grubby toenails—then you can kick off your shoes and show off your gorgeous feet.

Step-by-step nail care

Follow these easy steps to great looking toenails:

1. Start by washing your feet with warm, soapy water, then dry thoroughly with a clean towel, paying particular attention to the areas between your toes.

2. Gently wipe each toenail with a cotton wool pad dipped in a mild antiseptic, such as tea tree oil, which will remove any bacteria.

3. Massage cuticles with a cotton bud dipped in olive oil, and gently push them back with an orange stick.

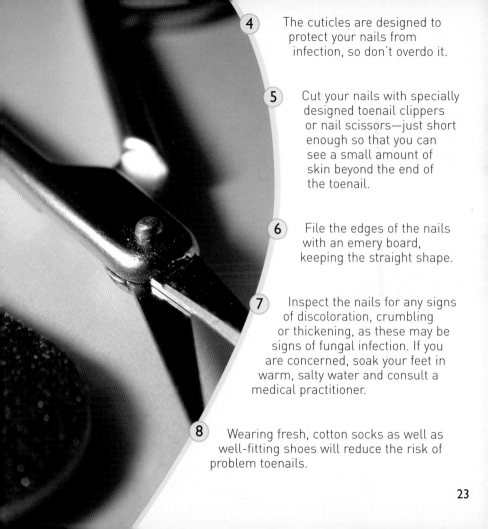

(4) The cuticles are designed to protect your nails from infection, so don't overdo it.

(5) Cut your nails with specially designed toenail clippers or nail scissors—just short enough so that you can see a small amount of skin beyond the end of the toenail.

(6) File the edges of the nails with an emery board, keeping the straight shape.

(7) Inspect the nails for any signs of discoloration, crumbling or thickening, as these may be signs of fungal infection. If you are concerned, soak your feet in warm, salty water and consult a medical practitioner.

(8) Wearing fresh, cotton socks as well as well-fitting shoes will reduce the risk of problem toenails.

23

Seeing a podiatrist

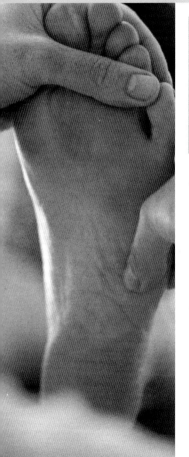

Chiropodists and podiatrists are people who are trained in the treatment of minor foot disorders. They should be qualified and registered by a professional body. The difference between a chiropodist and podiatrist is that a podiatrist will perform minor foot surgery, for example bunion operations, whereas a chiropodist does not.

Why visit?

Feet are a specialist area of the body and your doctor may not be the best person to diagnose and treat feet disorders. Chiropodists and podiatrists are trained to alleviate, prevent and treat disorders and give advice on proper foot care to patients.

A podiatrist or chiropodist can prevent, treat or advise on a variety of foot problems. Among the conditions and disorders that can be treated are fungal infections such as athlete's foot, muscle and joint pain, sprains, warts, ingrown toenails, bunions, hammertoes, and foot conditions caused by diabetes.

Treatments

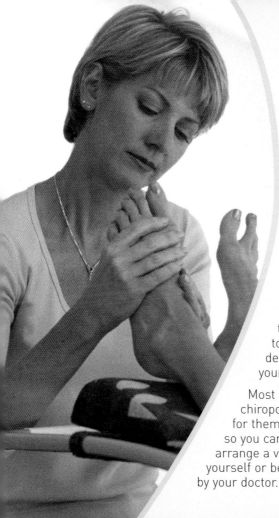

Podiatrists also make and fit orthotics (shoe inserts) after analyzing a patient's walk or run, and perform minor surgery under local anaesthetic. They work closely with other health care professionals to provide a comprehensive care plan for health problems.

If you suffer from any minor foot conditions, or more serious conditions such as diabetes or arthritis, a visit to a podiatrist may be well worthwhile. Some podiatrists specialize in surgery, sports injuries or foot disorders related to diabetes, so it may be valuable to seek them out, depending on your problem.

Most podiatrists and chiropodists work for themselves, so you can either arrange a visit yourself or be referred by your doctor.

Foot massage

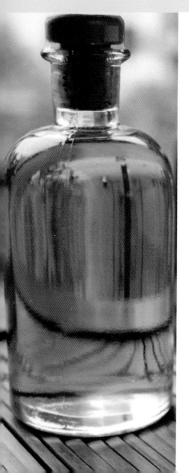

The relaxing and healing effects of foot massage have been recognized for thousands of years.

Drawings found in some tombs in Egypt show that foot massage was enjoyed by the ancient Egyptians.

In India and Thailand you can experience a foot massage in a department store. More and more people are turning to foot massage to counteract the stresses of modern-day life.

History of massage

The first recorded mention of massage is in an ancient Chinese text from 3000 years B.C. It became widely known when it was translated into French in the 1700s.

By 2500 B.C., the Egyptians had invented reflexology. The Indians created Ayurveda —a code of life that involves many massage techniques.

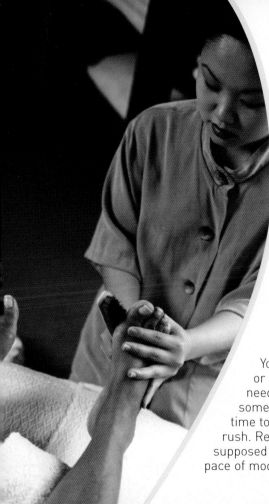

The Greeks were very keen on massage and many techniques we use today were first written down by them.

Massage continued to develop in the Far East. Western travelers often brought back word of the exotic and sensual massage techniques being practiced in these far-off lands.

A home massage

You don't have to visit a massage parlor to get a good massage. This is how you can give a wonderful foot massage to relieve tired, aching feet, or just for the sake of pampering!

You can either do it to yourself, or perform it on a friend. All you need is two or three fluffy towels, some lubricant and enough spare time to make sure you don't have to rush. Remember, a massage is supposed to be a break from the hectic pace of modern life!

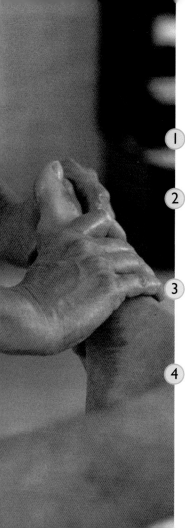

Step-by-step relaxation

You can use a base oil, such as sweet almond or jojoba oil, mixed with a few drops of your favorite essential oil, but any oil or rich cream will do.

1. Start by soaking the feet in warm water, then dry them thoroughly.

2. Place one foot on a towel and warm the oil or cream in your hands before gently massaging it over the whole foot, starting at the ankle and ending at the toes.

3. With your thumb, make gentle, circular movements over the sole of the foot, starting at the heel, pressing evenly and with no more pressure than is comfortable.

4. Place both hands around the foot, with fingers underneath and thumbs on the top of the foot. Gently move your thumb down the grooves between the tendons, working from the ankle to the toes.

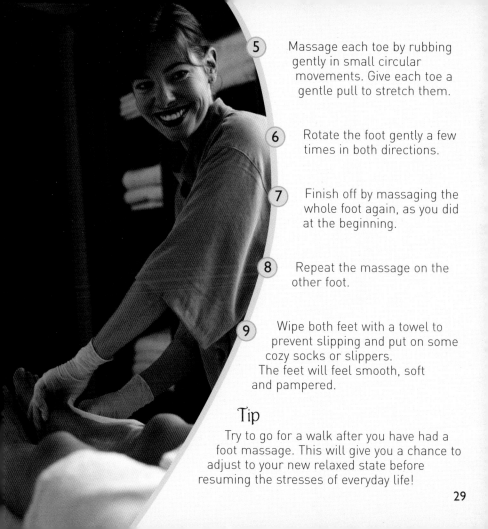

5. Massage each toe by rubbing gently in small circular movements. Give each toe a gentle pull to stretch them.

6. Rotate the foot gently a few times in both directions.

7. Finish off by massaging the whole foot again, as you did at the beginning.

8. Repeat the massage on the other foot.

9. Wipe both feet with a towel to prevent slipping and put on some cozy socks or slippers. The feet will feel smooth, soft and pampered.

Tip

Try to go for a walk after you have had a foot massage. This will give you a chance to adjust to your new relaxed state before resuming the stresses of everyday life!

Foot exercises

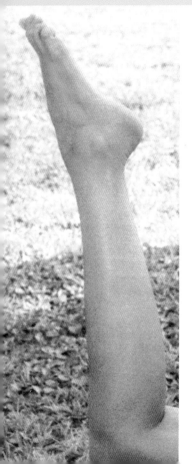

Just as the rest of your body needs exercise, so do your feet. Keeping your feet fit will strengthen and improve the flexibility of the muscles and joints.

Although walking is the best exercise for feet, there are times when we can't get out for a good walk.

The following simple exercises can be done almost anywhere—at home, or even sitting at your desk.

Ankle circles

Sit with your feet dangling above the floor. Rotate one foot from the ankle, first clockwise, then counterclockwise, repeating each movement five times. Repeat with the other foot.

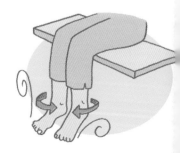

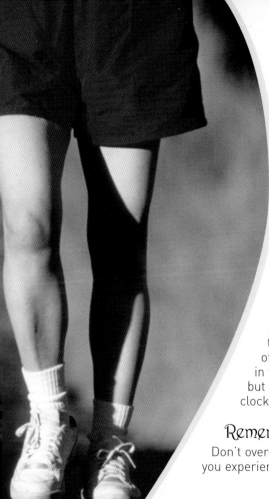

Foot raises

Sit with your feet flat on the floor. Raise the inner edge of one foot, so that the foot is resting on the outer edge. Curl your toes inward and hold for three seconds. Relax. Repeat ten times with each foot.

Foot circles

Sitting down, place your right foot flat on the floor, with your left in front of it with the heel down and toes pointing upwards. Circle the left foot in a counterclockwise direction ten times. Change the position of the feet, with the right foot in front. Repeat the exercise, but circle the right foot in a clockwise direction.

Remember

Don't overdo things at first and stop if you experience any pain or discomfort.

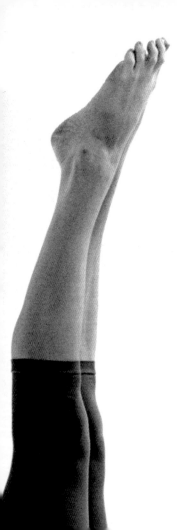

Ball rolls

Place a small ball, such as a tennis ball, under your foot and roll it for one to two minutes—hold onto the back of a chair for balance if you feel wobbly. This is excellent for massaging the bottom of your foot.

Toe lift

Sit with your feet flat on the floor. One foot at a time, keeping the rest of your foot still, lift your toes up as far as you can and hold for three seconds. Relax. Repeat ten times with each foot.

Marble pick-up

Not only is this a good exercise, but it can help you to clear up the room at the same time!

Place twenty marbles and an empty bowl on the floor. Use your toes to pick up the marbles and deposit them in the bowl.

Toe spreads

Place a thick rubber band around your toes and spread the toes for five seconds. Relax. Repeat ten times with each foot.

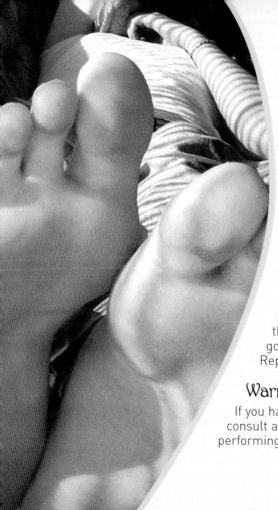

Toe curls

Sit with your feet dangling above the floor. Point one foot downward and curl your toes inwards. Hold for five seconds, then relax. Now pull the foot upwards and spread your toes out as far as possible. Hold for five seconds, then relax. Repeat ten times with each foot.

Toe wobbles

Sit with your toes extending over the edge of a smooth surface, such as a stair. Bend the toes downwards and hold for three seconds, then flex them upwards as far as they will go, holding for three seconds. Repeat ten times with each foot.

Warning

If you have any health or foot problems, consult a health care professional before performing these exercises.

Reflexology

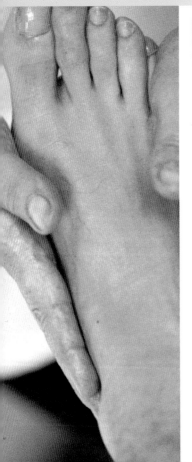

There are a number of complementary therapies available that can help you and your feet. Reflexology is one of them. It is an ancient technique that is growing in popularity.

What is reflexology?

Reflexology is a technique where pressure is applied to certain points on the feet that correspond to organs, glands and all parts of the body, to cure and prevent disease and promote well-being. This is achieved by applying pressure to specific tender spots that relate to problems elsewhere in the body.

According to reflexology, our bodies can heal themselves. Following illness, stress, injury or disease, the body is in a state of "imbalance" and vital energy pathways are blocked, preventing it functioning effectively. Reflexology can be used to restore and maintain the body's natural equilibrium and encourage healing.

For each person, the application and the effect of the therapy is unique.

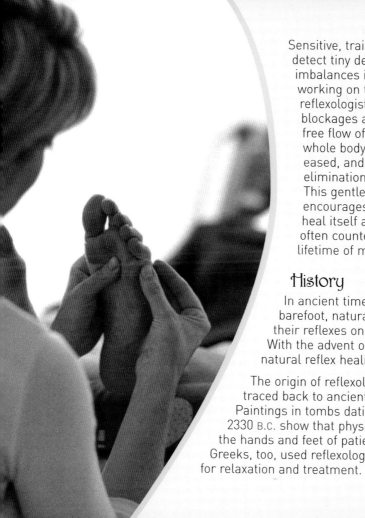

Sensitive, trained hands can detect tiny deposits and imbalances in the feet, and by working on these points the reflexologist can eliminate blockages and restore the free flow of energy to the whole body. Tensions are eased, and circulation and elimination is improved. This gentle therapy encourages the body to heal itself at its own pace, often counteracting a lifetime of misuse.

History

In ancient times people walked barefoot, naturally stimulating their reflexes on rough ground. With the advent of shoes, this natural reflex healing was lost.

The origin of reflexology can be traced back to ancient Egypt. Paintings in tombs dating back to 2330 B.C. show that physicians treated the hands and feet of patients. The ancient Greeks, too, used reflexology and massage for relaxation and treatment.

35

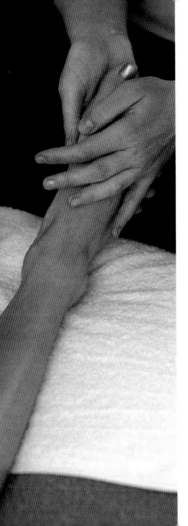

Modern reflexology

For many years reflexology remained unknown in the west as doctors concentrated on modern medicines and chemical cures. As people began to learn more about other parts of the world, and particularly their medicine, many forms of alternative therapy began to gain in popularity.

They were seen as practical alternatives to more conventional forms of health care, particularly by people concerned about using drugs to treat minor ailments. Modern reflexology has developed so that the whole body has been mapped onto the feet. Applying pressure to specific areas on the feet will have a reflex effect on the related part of the body.

The benefits

There are many benefits of reflexology. It aims to reduce stress and tension, cleanse the body of toxins, improve circulation, increase energy levels and encourage the body to heal naturally. A reflexology session will energize and revitalize you, leaving you feeling tingling and invigorated.

Regular sessions

Like most treatments, one session doesn't last forever so you will need to arrange for regular sessions to maintain the benefits.

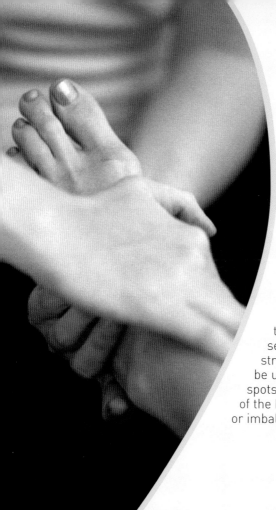

Warning!

Although reflexology is a
safe and easy method of
treatment, it should always
be performed by a qualified
reflexologist. It can be
beneficial for stress,
premenstrual tension,
fertility problems, cancer,
headaches and reducing
pain after surgery, among
other conditions.

What to expect

Sessions normally last about
an hour, with most of the
treatment concentrated on the
feet. Aromatherapy may be used
to help relaxation and focus the
senses. The pressure applied is
strong, but is not intended to
be uncomfortable, although tender
spots may indicate any areas
of the body that are congested
or imbalanced.

Pedicures

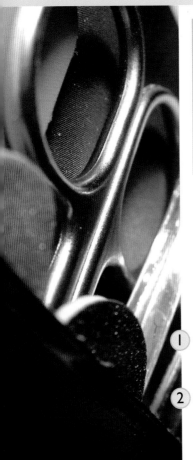

We all neglect our feet at times, especially during the winter months when they are constantly covered by socks, stockings and thick shoes. So it is often only when summer is just around the corner that we start to think about our feet, but any time is a good time to pamper them. A pedicure is not only a treat for your feet, it will leave you feeling relaxed, well-groomed and ready for anything.

You will need:

- a towel
- an orange stick
- an emery board
- moisturizer
- warm, soapy water
- nail clippers or nail scissors
- a pumice stone or foot file
- nail varnish

1. Wash your feet in warm, soapy water, giving them a good soak; then rinse them well.

2. Dry them thoroughly with a towel, paying particular attention to the area between the toes.

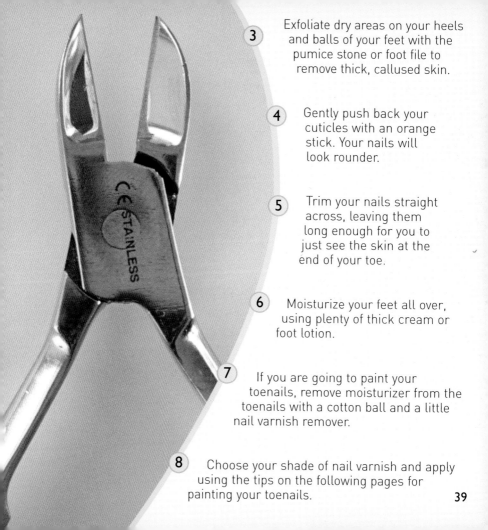

3 Exfoliate dry areas on your heels and balls of your feet with the pumice stone or foot file to remove thick, callused skin.

4 Gently push back your cuticles with an orange stick. Your nails will look rounder.

5 Trim your nails straight across, leaving them long enough for you to just see the skin at the end of your toe.

6 Moisturize your feet all over, using plenty of thick cream or foot lotion.

7 If you are going to paint your toenails, remove moisturizer from the toenails with a cotton ball and a little nail varnish remover.

8 Choose your shade of nail varnish and apply using the tips on the following pages for painting your toenails.

39

Pampering your feet

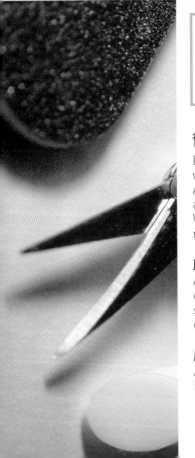

For fantastically fresh and pampered feet, why not try some of these homemade recipes that will leave your feet refreshed, smooth and soft. They are quick and easy to make and won't break the bank either.

Foot soaks

Look down the list of soaks on these pages to see which effects match how your feet are feeling. Add the ingredients to a large bowl of warm water and soak your feet for fifteen relaxing minutes. Why not pass the time catching up on some reading!

Lemon and cucumber

Add the juice of half a fresh lemon and half a cucumber, finely chopped. This is a refreshing soak and the lemon juice has a bleaching effect on yellowed nails.

Milk and honey

Add half a cup of milk and one tablespoon of honey for silky-feeling feet.

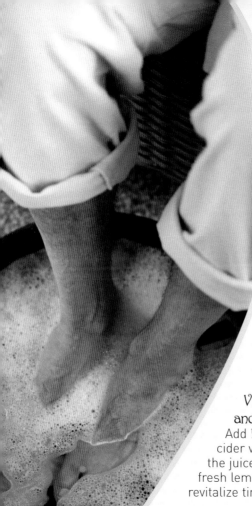

Vanilla oil
Two tablespoons of sweet almond oil and one teaspoon of pure vanilla extract will provide a smoothing and softening luxury soak.

Tea tree oil
Tea tree oil acts as an antiseptic. Two drops in the water is good for treating athlete's foot and toenail fungus infections.

Peppermint oil
Add two drops of peppermint oil to stimulate circulation and revive tired feet.

Epsom salts
Add ½ cup of Epsom salt. This soothes aching feet, softens rough skin and removes odors.

Vinegar and lemon
Add ½ cup of cider vinegar and the juice of half a fresh lemon to revitalize tired feet.

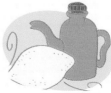

41

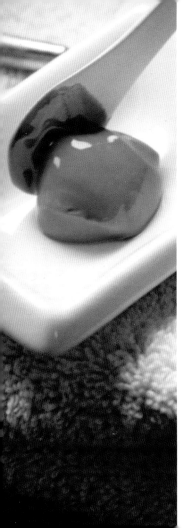

Foot scrubs

Sometimes a soak is just not enough. For extra silky-soft feet, an exfoliating foot scrub will help to remove dry, rough skin and dead skin cells. Remember to soak your feet for a few minutes to soften them before using the scrub.

Oatmeal and peppermint

To treat dry feet mix one tablespoon each of ground oatmeal and cornmeal and a teaspoon of salt in a small bowl. Add a little water, just enough to form a thick paste. Mix in two drops of peppermint oil. Massage into wet feet, scrubbing rough areas. Rinse well with warm water.

Almond and sugar

To soothe extra dry, rough feet, mix one tablespoon of sweet almond oil with two teaspoons of sugar. Add one teaspoon of honey and two or three drops of lavender oil. Mix well together and massage into wet feet. Rinse feet well with warm water.

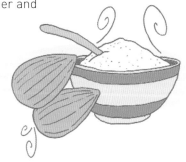

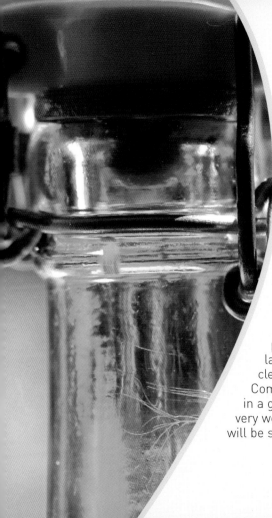

Foot moisturizers

Some days your feet are right up against it. A tough day can leave them feeling dry and worn out, so a wonderful, rich moisturizer is the ultimate pampering treatment.

Mix your own fragrant cream and enjoy the sensation of wonderfully moisturized feet.

Soothing

To make a soothing foot lotion, mix one tablespoon each of almond and olive oils, five drops of an essential oil, such as peppermint for aching feet, lavender for relaxing, or clementine for soothing. Combine the ingredients together in a glass bottle or jar and shake very well. Rub into your feet. They will be sure to thank you for it.

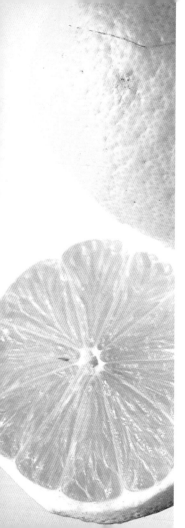

Softening

To make a softening foot lotion, mix one tablespoon each of jojoba and olive oils, and one teaspoon of vitamin E oil. Mix the ingredients together well. Rub into your feet, concentrating on any dry areas, such as the heels.

Moisturizing

For a moisturizing foot lotion, add together one tablespoon of olive oil, one teaspoon of honey, five drops of lemon juice and mix them well together. Rub into your feet and allow to dry thoroughly.

Warning!

Your feet may be slippery after applying these lotions, so it is advisable to wear socks until they have soaked into the skin completely.

Tip

It is important to moisturize your feet all year round. In summer we expose our feet to the harshness of the outdoors by going barefoot, and in winter the regenerative rate of skin slows, making it easier for the skin to dry out!

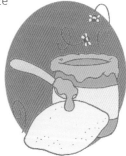

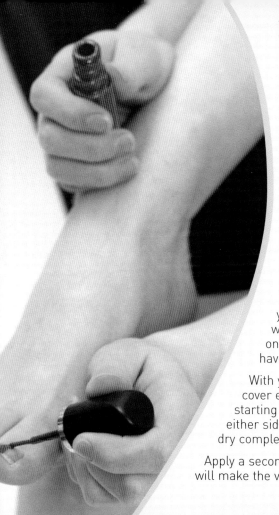

Painting your toenails

Now that your feet and toenails are looking great, finish off the look with a stunning color for super-sexy toes delicious enough to nibble!

A good idea
A toe separator will give you space between the toes and makes applying your varnish a lot easier and less messy.

Apply a basecoat, which will stop the varnish discoloring the nail. Allow to dry.

If your nails are already yellowed, soaking them in warm water with the juice of one lemon once a week will have a bleaching effect.

With your chosen varnish color, cover each nail in three strokes, starting in the center then painting on either side for an even coating. Allow to dry completely.

Apply a second coat over the first. Two coats will make the varnish last longer.

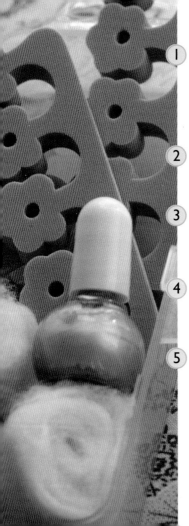

Step-by-step perfect toenails

1. When applying polish, don't have too much varnish on the brush, as this will make it more difficult to apply the varnish accurately and will leave the varnished nail looking and feeling "bumpy."

2. Leaving a slight gap on either side of the nail will make your toenails appear longer.

3. Apply a top coat to "seal" the varnish. If you are going to be in the sun, apply a top coat that has a sunscreen to stop your varnish fading.

4. Once the varnish is dry, carefully remove any excess varnish with a cotton bud soaked in nail varnish remover.

5. Allow the polish to dry completely before putting on closed-toe shoes.

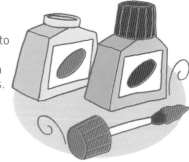

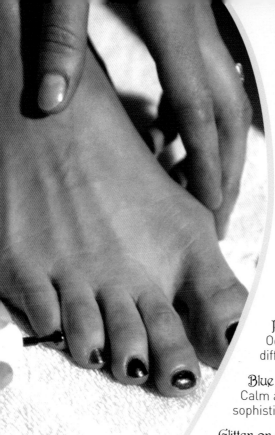

Color coordination

The range of colors available in modern nail varnishes is almost endless. While this may make choosing just the right color a mission in itself, it does mean that there is no excuse for sticking with boring red or claiming that you can't find just the right shade for you. Why not think about the following colors?

Red
If you want to stay with the perennial favorite, look out for the newer or unusual shades to give a contemporary feeling to your feet.

Purple
Oozes confidence—and a bit different. Step out in style.

Blue
Calm and serene—for a more sophisticated look.

Glitter or metallic
The ultimate party look. Guaranteed to make you want to get up and boogie!

Conclusion

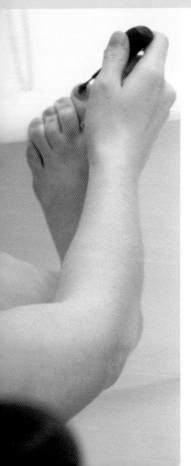

Reap the rewards

Your hard-working feet will reward you for keeping them healthy, beautiful and pampered by giving you many years of service. With feet fit for a princess you will want to show them off at any opportunity. This is also good for your feet, which hate being cooped up inside shoes all day, every day!

Spread the news

One of the best things about knowing how to look after your feet is sharing the knowledge with friends and family. Having friends round to share a soak, scrub or massage turns keeping your feet healthy into an enjoyable social occasion.

So, kick off your shoes, put your best foot forward and enjoy the huge number of benefits that healthy feet can bring.